Healthy Gourmet Wheat, Gluten, Dairy, Egg, and Yeast, Free Recipes

Dr. John A. Allocca

Copyright © 2014, 2019

Published by
Allocca Biotechnology, LLC
Northport, New York
www.allocca.com

ISBN 9781495999642

Healthy Gourmet Wheat, Gluten, Dairy, Egg, and Yeast, Free Recipes

Table of Contents

Other Books and Topics of Interest 6
    The Neurotransmitter Solution for Migraine, Depression, and more - Do It Yourself Guidebook 6
    Cookbook For The Mind 8
    Recipes Include: Brain Biofield Technology, Photography, Buddhism, Yoga, Shamanism 8

Brain Biofield Technology 11

Breakfast 14
    Almond Breakfast Cereal or Snack 14
    Cashew Breakfast Cereal or Snack 14

Appetizers 15
    Baba Ghannouj 15
    Bean Dip 16
    Bean Salad 16
    Hummus 17
    Indian Red Relish 18
    Salmon Spread 18

Soups 19

Healthy Gourmet Wheat, Gluten, Dairy, Egg, and Yeast, Free Recipes

    Bean and Mushroom Soup 19
    Vegetable Soup 20
    Spaghetti Squash Soup 21

Snacks 22
    Zucchini 22
    Mushrooms 22
    Vegetables 23

Sauces 23
    Curry Sauce 23
    Marinara Sauce 24
    Garlic and Oil Sauce 25
    Pesto Sauce 25
    Tahini Sauce & Dressing 26
    Tomato Sauce 26

Main Dishes 27

Baked Tilapia 27
Bok Choy and Mushrooms 28
Broiled Salmon 28
Chicken Creole 29
Blackened Tuna...30
Chicken Cacciatore 31
Chicken Casserole with Crushed Tomatoes..........32
Chili 33
Chopped Meat (Turkey) Allocca Style 34
Curry Casserole 35
Easy Dinner...36
Healthy Salad 37
Kale Casserole 37
Meat (Turkey) Loaf 38
Portobella Casserole 39
Roasted Chicken 40
Sausage (Chicken) with Onions and Peppers 41
Stuffed Chicken with Mushrooms..........................42
Stuffed Chicken with Tomatoes and Olives 43
Turkey 44
Vegetable Casserole 45

Side Dishes **46**

    Baked French Fries 46
    Broccoli with Tomato Sauce 47
    Dahl 47
    Lentil Salad 48
    Mushrooms in Garlic & Oil 49
    Oil and Lemon Dressing 49
    Squash 50
    Steamed Vegetables 51
    Stuffed Artichokes 52
    Tossed Salad 52

Bread and Muffins 53
    Banana Nut Muffins 53
    Blueberry Muffins 54
    Brown Rice Bread 55
    Brown Rice Foccacia Bread 56
    Corn Muffins 57

Desserts 58
    Almond Cookies and Pancakes 58
    Apple Cashew Dessert 59
    Carrot Cake 60
    Carob or Chocolate Brownies or Cake 61
    Cashew Cookies and Pancakes 62
    Coconut Icing 63
    Pie Crust 63
    Pie Filling - Apple 64
    Pie Filling - Blueberry 64
    Pumpkin Pudding or Pie Filling 65

Healthy Gourmet Wheat, Gluten, Dairy, Egg, and Yeast, Free Recipes

Other Books and Topics of Interest

The Neurotransmitter Solution for Migraine, Depression, and more - Do It Yourself Guidebook

John A. Allocca, D.Sc., Ph.D. Copyright 2019
ISBN-13: 978-1082175763
136 - 6" x 9" pages

There are three options here. Do it yourself, get professional help, or both. For most people, the guidelines herein will be adequate. If there are complications, help may be needed. Allocca Biotechnology, LLC offers a customized program based on test results. This is available at www.allocca.com. The customized assessment can be done via mail, email, and phone. In either case, the steps in this book are the best way to start.

The loss of neurotransmitters cause other problems such as, Migraine Headaches, Depression, Insomnia, Anger, Violence, and Bipolar Syndrome, Decreased Sexuality, Increased Appetite for Carbohydrates, Irritable Bowel Syndrome, Tinnitus, Fibromyalgia, Premenstrual Syndrome (PMS), and Seasonal Affective Disorder (SAD). Imbalances of serotonin and norepinephrine affect your body and behavior.

Table of Contents:

The Author's Journey with Migraine

Do it Yourself or Get Help

Step 1 - Understanding Migraine and Other Neurotransmitter Disorders

Step 2 - Eliminate the Offenders

Step 3 - Hydration

Step 4 - Neurobiology Formula 121397 (NeuroLife)

Step 5 - Stress Reduction with BrainicityTM E.L.F. Brain Biofield Therapy

Step 6 - Stress Reduction with Desktop Yoga

Step 7 - Fine Tuning with Gluten and Dairy

Step 8 - Fine Tuning with Caffeine

Step 9 - Fine Tuning with The Glycemic Index

Step 10 - Fun with Wheat, Gluten, Dairy, Egg, and Yeast, Free Recipes

Step 11 - Other Suggested Reading and Fun

Order printed book from Amazon

Order kindle book from Amazon

Healthy Gourmet Wheat, Gluten, Dairy, Egg, and Yeast, Free Recipes

Cookbook For The Mind
Recipes Include: Brain Biofield Technology, Photography, Buddhism, Yoga, Shamanism

Dr. John A. Allocca, Copyright 2019
ISBN 9781691698615
182 - 6" x 9" pages

Everyone wants inner peace. It is the lack of inner peace that causes hatred and violence. For thousands of years various disciplines have structured long studies, mentoring, and meditations of some sort to achieve the goal of inner peace. Most of these disciplines are found in eastern cultures. The fast-paced western society has shown little interest in them, with some small exceptions. What is the solution? The solution or part of the solution is to develop a methodology that comprises of technology and some aspects of the various disciplines that will be useful and of interest to people in western society.

Almost everyone in western society has a cell phone with a camera, which makes photography easy. Photography is a tool used in this methodology to to explore what people feel inside. Any camera or cell phone can be used. What are you called to photograph? What emotions does the photograph bring to the surface? How does it make you feel? This book will help to guide you through this process.

This book contains two of Dr. Allocca's personal journeys: 2009 and 2018.

Mindfulness and control of Ego Control Battles are another tool that is used to understand and improve interactions with others.

Brain biofield technology is used in this methodology to calm the mind and develop interactions between the left and right hemispheres of the brain. Or, one can use meditation or both.

For the body and the mind is "Desktop Yoga." This is a methodology that requires little time and little effort. It was developed for those in a rush or for those with little energy.

Last, but not least, no cookbook will be complete without dessert. Gluten free desserts are included in this book for pleasure.

Dr. Allocca is a medical research scientist and biophysicist with many years of personal experience in photography and with some knowledge of Buddhism, Shamanism, and Yoga.

Table of Contents:
   Introduction
   Awakening
   Consciousness

Mindfulness and Ego Control Battles
A Dash of Buddhism
Brain Biofield Technology
The Genesis Meditation
A Dash of Yoga
The Journey Started in Sedona
A Dash of Shamanism (Vision Quest Journey)
Vision Quest - East 2009
Vision Quest - South 2009
Vision Quest - West 2009
Vision Quest - North 2009
Vision Quest - East 2018
Vision Quest - South 2018
Vision Quest - West 2018
Vision Quest - North 2018
Your Personal Journey Guidance - Part 1 - Beginning with a Camera
Your Personal Journey Guidance - Part 2 - Beginning Assignments
Your Personal Journey Guidance - Part 3 - East
Your Personal Journey Guidance - Part 4 - South
Your Personal Journey Guidance - Part 5 - West
Your Personal Journey Guidance - Part 6 - North
Your Personal Journey Guidance - Part 7 - Journey Reflection
Gluten Free Desserts

Order the full color printed book from Amazon
Order the color Kindle ebook from Amazon

Healthy Gourmet Wheat, Gluten, Dairy, Egg, and Yeast, Free Recipes

Brain Biofield Technology

Make Your Brain Happy

Brainicty™ Brain Biofield Therapy uses Integrated Harmonic Wave Audio Patterns to:
- Reduce Stress and Anxiety
- Reduce Attention Deficit
- Reduce Headaches
- Reduce Phobias
- Reduce P.T.S.D.
- Help with Epilepsy
- Increase Cognitive Function
- Get Better Sleep
- Increase Performance

The heart produces electromagnetic signals, which may be called electrocardiography (ECG) or the heart biofield. The brain produces electromagnetic signals, which may be called electroencephalography (EEG) or the brain biofield. The brain produces an erratic biofield that can be deciphered. Brain waves are classified by frequencies as Delta, Theta, Alpha, and Beta waves. Delta (0.5 Hz to 4 Hz) is seen normally in slow wave sleep. Theta (4 Hz to 8 Hz) is seen in drowsiness, meditation, and creative states. Alpha (5 Hz to 12 Hz) emerges with closing of the eyes and with relaxation, and attenuates with eye opening or mental exertion. Beta (12 Hz to 30 Hz) is associated with active, busy or anxious thinking and active concentration.

Brainicity™ uses integrated harmonic wave audio patterns to facilitate multiple brain biofield resonances. A sine wave would produce an infinite number of even harmonics. A square wave would produce an infinite number of odd harmonics. Too many harmonics can cause the brain to be overwhelmed because it has a limit of how much information can be processed at a given time resulting in the brain ignoring the inputs. Too little harmonics will not be effective. An integrated wave will produce a limited number of harmonics, which can be interpreted by the brain.

Resonance occurs when the frequency of a periodic waveform is in phase with an external periodic waveform of equal or almost equal frequency to the internal frequency. This causes the system to oscillate with a larger amplitude than the force applied at other frequencies. Waveforms in the frequency range of 0.5 to 20 hertz are below the human hearing range. In order for the brain to be able to sense brain wave frequencies it cannot hear, the difference between two frequencies within the human hearing range is used to produce a third frequency within the brain wave frequencies (brain biofield). Then, that resulting complex pattern of waveforms are set to achieve multiple resonances with the brain's own waves.

In a clinical study, the Brainicty™ system caused an immediate increase in alpha brain waves.

The BrainicityTM system is designed to be used with speakers or headphones. It also includes a musical background to make the experience more pleasurable.

It is simple to use. Listen to one track just before bedtime for a good nights sleep. Dim the lights. Then, just sit back and relax for 21 minutes.

Use STEREO headphones or earphones only.

The Brainicty™ (NeuroPath2) Efficacy Study 2015-2016, indicated there was a 51% decrease in anxiety, 36% increase in ability to sleep, 34% increase in ability to remember dreams, 43% reduction in pain, 35% increase in ability to cope with stress, and 41% increase in ability to focus. There was a positive effect after treatment in all parameters. There were no foreseeable adverse side effects that can be imagined or were experienced in this study.

Visit www.allocca.com for more information.

Healthy Gourmet Wheat, Gluten, Dairy, Egg, and Yeast, Free Recipes

Breakfast

Almond Breakfast Cereal or Snack

1/4 cup almond flour
1/4 cup cashew nuts, chopped coarsely
1/4 teaspoon ground cinnamon
Dash of nutmeg
1/8 cup water

Cashew Breakfast Cereal or Snack

1/4 cup almond flour
1/4 cup cashew nuts, chopped coarsely
1/4 teaspoon ground cinnamon
Dash of nutmeg
1/8 cup water

Healthy Gourmet Wheat, Gluten, Dairy, Egg, and Yeast, Free Recipes

Appetizers

Baba Ghannouj

Preheat oven to 450 degrees F.
2 large eggplants (about 2 pounds)
1/4 cup lemon juice (not for migraineur's)
3 tablespoons cold pressed sesame oil
2 cloves garlic, finely mashed
4 tablespoons sesame seeds
1/2 teaspoon sea salt
1/2 teaspoon black pepper

Peel and grate the eggplants. Bake grated eggplant in a casserole with cover for 45 minutes. Remove from oven and let stand until cool. Simmer garlic in oil a few minutes or until lightly brown. Mix all ingredients with an electric mixer for 1 minute. Place mixture in a bowl, cover and refrigerate for one day. Remove from refrigerator 30 minutes before serving. Serve with vegetables you like except potatoes or carrots

Bean Dip
3 tablespoons cold pressed olive or sunflower oil
2 cloves garlic, chopped
30 oz. refried beans
3/4 cup water
1/2 teaspoon basil
1/4 teaspoon black pepper
1/2 teaspoon oregano
1/2 teaspoon parsley
1/2 teaspoon sea salt

    Using a deep skillet, sauté the garlic in olive or sunflower oil until dark brown. Lower heat and add remaining ingredients. Cook for another 5 minutes. Serve with vegetables you like except potatoes or carrots

Bean Salad
16 oz. kidney beans or white beans, drained
16 oz. garbanzo beans, drained
Olive or sunflower oil to taste
Garlic powder to taste
Oregano to taste
Chives to taste

    Mix the above ingredients together and serve.

Hummus

16 oz. garbanzo beans
3 tablespoons cold pressed olive or sunflower oil
1 clove garlic or more, finely mashed
1 teaspoon parsley
3 tablespoons lemon juice (not for migraineur's)
dash of cayenne pepper
1/4 cup water

Add garbanzo beans, sesame oil, garlic, lemon juice, cayenne, and 1/4 cup of water to a food processor. Process until smooth. Add more water if mixture is too thick. Allow to chill in the refrigerator for at least one hour. Spread on a flat platter and garnish with parley. Serve with vegetables you like except potatoes or carrots.

Indian Red Relish

2 cloves garlic, chopped
1 onion, chopped (optional)
8 oz. tomato puree
3 tablespoons cold pressed olive or sunflower oil
1/2 teaspoon cayenne pepper or less
1 teaspoon turmeric
1/2 teaspoon coriander
1/2 teaspoon cumin
1/4 teaspoon salt
1/4 teaspoon black pepper
1 tablespoon lemon juice (not for migraineur's)
1/4 cup water

Mix all above ingredients. Serve with vegetables you like except potatoes or carrots.

Salmon Spread

1/2 pound salmon, cooked
3 teaspoons cold pressed olive or sunflower oil
1/8 teaspoon cayenne pepper
1/2 teaspoon basil
1/4 cup lemon juice (not for migraineur's)
1/4 teaspoon sea salt
1/8 teaspoon black pepper

Blend salmon in food processor. Gradually add oil. Add the remaining ingredients and continue blending until mixture is smooth. Cover and store in refrigerator. Serve chilled.

Soups

Bean and Mushroom Soup

4 tablespoons cold pressed olive or sunflower oil
2 large cloves garlic, chopped
1/2 tablespoon organic butter
1 bunch scallions, chopped
3/4 pound mushrooms, sliced
4 cups water
1/2 teaspoon sea salt
1/2 teaspoon black pepper
Dash of cayenne pepper
1 tablespoon parsley
1 tablespoon basil
1 tablespoon oregano
2 cans white beans, drained and washed

In a 6-quart pot, sauté the garlic, olive or sunflower oil, and butter at medium heat until the garlic is lightly brown. Add the scallions and continue to cook for another minute. Add the mushrooms and continue cooking for another 5 minutes. Add the remaining ingredients and simmer for 20 minutes. Remove the pot from the stove and puree the soup with a hand blender. Caution soup is hot. Be very careful while pureeing. Serve hot.

Vegetable Soup
8 cups water (3 quarts)
1 cup brown or green lentils
1 pound mushrooms, sliced
4 stalks celery, sliced
2 cloves garlic, chopped
2 tablespoons parsley
2 teaspoon basil
1/8 teaspoon or more cayenne pepper
1/2 teaspoon black pepper
1 teaspoon sea salt

     Bring water to a boil in an 8-quart pot. Add ingredients and allow to a boil for 3 minutes. Lower heat and simmer for 1 hour. Stir occasionally. Serve hot. Leftover soup can be frozen. Serves 6 to 8 people.

Spaghetti Squash Soup

3 tablespoons cold pressed olive or sunflower oil
2 cloves garlic, chopped
1 spaghetti squash
Chinese cabbage or bok choy (optional)
1 red bell pepper, chopped
1 green bell pepper, chopped
1 onion, chopped (optional)
1/2 pound mushroom, sliced
1 teaspoon sea salt
1/2 teaspoon black pepper
1 teaspoon parsley
1 teaspoon basil
1/2 teaspoon oregano
1/8 teaspoon or more cayenne pepper
Water

    Bake the spaghetti squash in an over for 1 hour at 375 degrees F. Remove it from the oven and allow it to cool. Cut the squash in half lengthwise. Remove the seeds. With a fork, strip the strands of squash from the shell.

    Sauté garlic in olive or sunflower oil until lightly brown in an 8-quart pot at medium heat. Add onions, peppers and mushrooms. Continue cooking for about 5 minutes. Add the remaining ingredients. Add water to about 1 inch above the ingredients. Cook for 1 hour at low heat.

Snacks

Zucchini

1 raw zucchini
Cold pressed olive or sunflower oil
Sea salt
Black pepper
Oregano

Skin the zucchini. Cut it into slices that are about 1/4 inch thick. Lay them out on a plate. Add a few drops of olive or sunflower oil and other ingredients on top of each. Serve cold.

Mushrooms

Raw button mushrooms
Cold pressed olive or sunflower oil
Sea salt
Black pepper
Oregano

Cut in half. Lay them out on a plate with the cut side up. Add a few drops of olive or sunflower oil and other ingredients on top of each. Serve cold.

Vegetables

Any raw vegetables you like except potatoes or carrots
Cold pressed olive or sunflower oil
Sea salt
Black pepper
Oregano

Cut the vegetables as desired. Lay them out on a plate. Add a few drops of olive or sunflower oil and other ingredients on top of each. Serve cold.

Sauces

Curry Sauce

3 tablespoons cold pressed olive or sunflower oil
2 cloves garlic, chopped
16 oz. tomato puree
1/2 teaspoon black pepper
1/2 teaspoon cardamom
A dash or more of cayenne
1 teaspoon turmeric
1/2 teaspoon coriander
1/2 teaspoon cumin
1/4 teaspoon sea salt

Sauté garlic and oil in a 3-quart pot. Add remaining ingredients. Simmer for 10 to 20 minutes.

Marinara Sauce

3 tablespoons cold pressed olive or sunflower oil
4 large cloves garlic, chopped
1 onion, chopped (optional)
28 oz. whole tomatoes
6 fresh basil leaves, chopped
1 tablespoon oregano
1 tablespoon parsley
1 tablespoon basil
1/2 teaspoon sea salt
1/2 teaspoon black pepper
Dash of cayenne pepper

    The origins of marinara sauce, is that the sauce was made in Naples for the sailors when they returned from the sea. The sauce does not contain fish or anything from the sea.

    In an 6-quart pot, sauté' garlic and olive or sunflower oil at medium heat until the garlic is soft and lightly browned. Crush the tomatoes with a fork or puree the tomatoes in a blender. Add remaining ingredients except the basil. Bring to a boil, then lower heat to a simmer and cook until thickened approximately 20 to 30 minutes. Add basil just before serving. Serve over vegetables. Serves 2-4 people.

Garlic and Oil Sauce

3 tablespoons cold pressed olive or sunflower oil
2 cloves garlic, finely chopped
1 teaspoon parsley
1/2 teaspoon oregano
1/2 teaspoon sea salt
1/8 teaspoon black pepper
1/4 cup soup broth

     Sauté garlic until brown; let cool for 2 minutes. Add rest of ingredients and continue cooking for 5-10 minutes. Add vegetables.

Pesto Sauce

2 cups fresh basil leaves
1 cup parsley
1/4 cup cold pressed olive or sunflower oil
2 cloves garlic, pressed

     Mix in a food processor or blender, heat mildly and pour over 1/2 to 1 pound of brown rice or quinoa pasta. Serves 2 people.

Tahini Sauce & Dressing

1 cup sesame tahini
1/2 cup or more water
4 tablespoons lemon juice (not for migraineur's)
4 tablespoons cold pressed olive or sunflower oil
1/2 teaspoon sea salt
1/2 teaspoon black pepper

    Mix above ingredients in a blender until smooth. If used as a salad dressing, add more water.

Tomato Sauce

4 tablespoons cold pressed olive or sunflower oil
2 cloves garlic, chopped
2 onions, chopped (optional)
32 oz. tomato puree
1/2 pound mushrooms, sliced
1 tablespoon oregano
1 tablespoon fresh basil
1 tablespoon parsley
1/2 tablespoon sea salt
1/2 teaspoon black pepper
1/2 teaspoon or less cayenne pepper
6 fresh basil leaves, chopped
1 pound any vegetables you like except potatoes or carrots

    In an 8-quart pot sauté garlic in oil until brown. Add remaining ingredients. Simmer 2 hours, stirring every 15 minutes. Serves over vegetables.

Main Dishes

Baked Tilapia

Preheat oven to 350 degrees F.
Fresh tilapia
Cold pressed olive or sunflower oil
Sea salt
Black pepper
Garlic powder
Oregano

Add a little olive or sunflower oil to the bottom of a 24-ounce au gratin baking dish or a Pyrex 9.5 x 15.2 x 2.2 inch baking dish. Place the tilapia (3 tilapia in the Pyrex dish) with the side with the red marks, down into the baking dish. Sprinkle some olive or sunflower oil over the tilapia. Sprinkle some salt, pepper, garlic powder and oregano over the top of the tilapia. Cover with aluminum foil. Bake in the oven at 350 degrees F for 30 minutes. Each tilapia feeds one.

Bok Choy and Mushrooms

1 pound mushrooms, sliced
1 head of bok choy, cut up
2 tablespoons butter
Cold pressed olive or sunflower oil
Oregano
2 tablespoons butter

Add butter to a skillet at medium heat. When butter melts, add the mushrooms. When mushrooms are browned, add the boy choy and cook until boy choy is fully cooked.

Remove from heat and add olive or sunflower oil and oregano.

Serve over rice.

Broiled Salmon

Salmon (4-6 oz per person)
Pepper
Garlic Powder
Oregano

Place the salmon with the skin down in a foil tray and add oregano. Broil at 400 degrees F for 20 minutes. Remove from toaster oven and add pepper, garlic powder, and oregano. Remove from the foil pan. The skin should stick to the bottom of the pan.

Serve with rice and vegetables

Chicken Creole

3 tablespoons cold pressed olive or sunflower oil
3 cloves garlic, chopped
2 cloves of garlic, chopped
1 green pepper, chopped
2 pounds chicken breasts, cut into 3/4" pieces
2 stalks of celery, diced
1 large bay leaf
1 teaspoon basil
1/8 teaspoon black pepper
1/8 teaspoon cayenne pepper
1 teaspoon parsley
1/2 teaspoon sea salt
16 oz. tomato puree
2 cups water

    Heat oil (high-medium) in deep sauté pan. Sauté garlic for 10 minutes or until brown. Add garlic and green pepper, and continue cooking for another 5 minutes. Add all other ingredients and continue cooking for 10 minutes. Serves 2 to 4 people.

Blackened Tuna

2 tuna filets or steaks
3 tablespoons cold pressed olive or sunflower oil
2 cloves garlic, chopped
1 teaspoon or more black pepper
1 teaspoon parsley
3 oz. baby spinach

Place the olive or sunflower oil in a large sauté' pan at medium-high heat. Add the garlic and cook until slightly brown. Push the garlic to the edge around the pan. Add black pepper to both sides of the tuna. Place the tuna in the center of the pan. Add the other spices to everything in the pan. Cook the tuna until it is browned. Turn over and brown the other side. The tuna is done when the center is cooked. Serve over a bed of spinach. Serves two.

Chicken Cacciatore

3 tablespoons cold pressed olive or sunflower oil
2 cloves garlic, chopped
1 onion, chopped (optional)
32 oz. tomato puree
1 whole chicken cut up in pieces
1 tablespoon oregano
1 tablespoon parsley
1/2 tablespoon sea salt
1/4 teaspoon black pepper
2 basil leaves
1 pound any vegetables you like except potatoes or carrots

    Brown garlic in oil in a small fry pan. Put all ingredients together in an 8-quart pot. Simmer 1 hour, stirring every 15 minutes. Serves 4 people.

Chicken Casserole with Crushed Tomatoes

Preheat oven to 350 degrees F.
3 pounds thin sliced chicken breast (about 6 pieces)
2 cloves garlic, finely chopped
28 oz organic crushed plum tomatoes
3 tablespoons Cold pressed olive or sunflower oil
1/4 teaspoon sea salt
1/8 teaspoon fine black pepper
1 teaspoon parsley
6 fresh basil leaves, chopped
1 teaspoon oregano
Dash of cayenne pepper (optional)

    Mix the above ingredients, except the chicken, in a bowl. Place a small amount of olive or sunflower oil on the bottom of a covered Pyrex baking dish. Place the chicken breasts on the bottom of the dish. Pour over some tomato mixture. Add another layer of chicken breasts. Pour over more tomato mixture. Pour the remaining tomato mixture on the top layer. Cover and bake 90 minutes at 350 degrees F. Serves 6 people.

Chili

3 tablespoons cold pressed olive or sunflower oil
2 cloves garlic, finely chopped
1 onion, chopped (optional)
1 green pepper, chopped
16 oz. tomatoes, finely chopped
16 oz. tomato puree
16 oz. white beans, drained
1 cup water
1 teaspoon basil
1/2 teaspoon black pepper
6 teaspoons chili powder
1 teaspoon oregano
1 teaspoon parsley
1/2 teaspoon sea salt

    Heat oil in an 8-quart pot at medium heat. Sauté garlic, and peppers until brown. Add remaining ingredients. Cover and simmer for 60 minutes. Add more water if sauce is too thick. Serves 6 people.

Chopped Meat (Turkey) Allocca Style

2 tablespoons cold pressed olive or sunflower oil
2 cloves garlic, chopped
1 onion, chopped (optional)
1/2 green pepper, finely chopped
16 oz. tomato puree
1 pound chopped turkey
1 teaspoon oregano
1/2 teaspoon parsley
1/2 teaspoon basil
1/2 teaspoon garlic powder
1/2 teaspoon sea salt
1/8 teaspoon black pepper
Dash cayenne pepper

Sauté garlic. Place remaining ingredients in a 4-quart pot, cover and cook for 10 -15 minutes over a medium heat, stirring frequently. Serve hot. Serves 2 people.

Curry Casserole

3 tablespoons cold pressed olive or sunflower oil
2 cloves garlic, chopped
1 onion, chopped (optional)
16 oz. tomato puree
16 oz. lentils
1 head broccoli, chopped
1/2 teaspoon sea salt
1/2 teaspoon black pepper
1/2 teaspoon cardamom
A dash of cayenne, to your taste
1 teaspoon turmeric
1/2 teaspoon coriander
1/2 teaspoon cumin

     In a 6-quart pot, sauté garlic in oil until slightly brown. Add rice and sauté for another minute. Add remaining ingredients. Bring to a boil. Cover, lower heat, and simmer for 45 minutes.

Easy Dinner

Place your favorite vegetables into a corning ware casserole.
Add a small amount of butter.
Cover and cook in microwave for 10 minutes
Remove cover and add olive oil or sunflower oil, pepper, garlic powder, and oregano.
Mix with wooden spoon.

In a foil oven pan, add one piece of wild salmon with the skin facing down
Broil in toaster oven for 20 minutes
Remove from toaster oven and add pepper, garlic powder, and oregano.
Remove from the foil pan. The skin should stick to the bottom of the pan.

Serve with salad or rice.

Healthy Salad

Romaine lettuce

Spinach

Cabbage, sliced

Red or green pepper, cut up

Bean sprouts

Mushrooms, sliced

Any additional vegetables you like except potatoes or carrots

Kale Casserole

2 tablespoons cold pressed olive or sunflower oil

2 cloves garlic, chopped

1 onion, chopped (optional)

1 large bunch of kale, chopped

1 tablespoon lemon juice (not for migraineur's)

1/2 teaspoon sea salt

1/4 teaspoon black pepper

1 teaspoon basil

1/2 teaspoon parsley

1/2 teaspoon oregano

     In a 6-quart pot, sauté garlic in oil until slightly brown. Add rice and sauté for another minute. Add remaining ingredients. Bring to a boil. Cover, lower heat, and simmer for 45 minutes.

Meat (Turkey) Loaf

Preheat oven to 425 degrees F.
2 tablespoons cold pressed olive or sunflower oil
2 cloves garlic, chopped
1 onion, chopped (optional)
1 green pepper, chopped
1/2 pound fresh mushrooms, sliced
8 oz. tomato puree
2 pounds lean chopped turkey
1 tablespoon oregano
1/2 teaspoon parsley
1/2 teaspoon black pepper
1/2 teaspoon basil
1/2 teaspoon sea salt
2 teaspoons xantham gum
1/2 teaspoon agar agar

Sauté garlic till brown and put aside. Sauté mushrooms till brown and put aside. Mix all above ingredients except tomato sauce. Make into a load and cover with tomato sauce. Bake in oven at 425 degrees for 60 minutes. Serves 2 to 4 people

Portobella Casserole
2 tablespoons cold pressed olive or sunflower oil or more
2 cloves garlic, chopped
1 onion, chopped (optional)
1 pound Portabella mushrooms, diced into 3/4" squares
3-1/2 cups water
6 oz. baby spinach
1/2 teaspoon sea salt
1/4 teaspoon black pepper
1 teaspoon basil
1/2 teaspoon parsley
1/2 teaspoon oregano

In a 6-quart pot, sauté garlic in oil until slightly brown. Add mushrooms and sauté for another 5 minutes. Add rice and sauté for another minute. Add remaining ingredients. Bring to a boil. Cover, lower heat, and simmer for 45 minutes.

Roasted Chicken

Preheat oven to 350 degrees F.

Oil the bottom of a large poultry pan with v-shaped rack. Place cut potatoes and carrots on the bottom of the pan. Place cut onions and carrots on top of the potatoes. Sprinkle with cold pressed olive or sunflower oil, sea salt (small amount), black pepper, parsley, basil, and oregano. Place the chicken on the v-shaped rack. Approximate cooking times (20 minutes per pound plus an additional 20 minutes):

    3 pounds = 1 hour, 20 minutes
    3.5 pounds = 1 hour, 30 minutes
    4 pounds = 1 hour, 40 minutes
    5 pounds = 2 hours
    6 pounds = 2 hours, 20 minutes
    7 pounds = 2 hours, 40 minutes
    8 pounds = 3 hours minutes

Note: if two chickens are used, calculate the time for the weight of the larger chicken and add 30 minutes.

Note: if the chicken(s) were frozen and not fully thawed, add 30 minutes to the cooking time.

The roasting pan recommended is the "Rachael Ray Oven Lovin' Non-Stick 10" x 14" Roaster with V-Rack." The non-stock pan and rack make it is easy to clean. Two 3.5 pound chickens can fit in this pan.

Sausage (Chicken) with Onions and Peppers

2 pounds chicken sausage
2 tablespoons cold pressed olive or sunflower oil
2 onions, chopped
2 bell peppers, chopped
1 teaspoon parsley
1 teaspoon oregano
1 teaspoon basil
1/2 teaspoon sea salt
1/8 teaspoon black pepper

In a 6-quart pot, add the oil, onions, and peppers. Cook covered over medium heat for 5 minutes. Add the sausages and continue cooking covered for 20 minutes or until done. Serves 2 to 4 people.

Stuffed Chicken with Mushrooms

1 pound portabella or button mushrooms, chopped
2 tablespoons cold pressed olive or sunflower oil
1/2 teaspoon sea salt
1/4 teaspoon black pepper
Dash of cayenne pepper
1/2 teaspoon parsley
1/2 teaspoon basil
1/2 teaspoon oregano
2 cloves garlic, chopped
1 onion, chopped (optional)
3 pounds (10 slices) thin-sliced chicken breast

Sauté mushrooms in oil for 5 minutes. Add herbs and spices and set aside. Place 5 thin-sliced chicken breasts into an oiled 15 x 10 x 2 Pyrex dish. Add some mushroom mixture to each slice. Next, place another 5 thin-sliced chicken breast on top of each of the previously filled breasts. Add the remaining mixture on top of each thin-sliced chicken breast. Place in the oven and low broil for 35 minutes.

Stuffed Chicken with Tomatoes and Olives

16 oz tomato puree
16 oz black olives, chopped
2 tablespoons cold pressed olive or sunflower oil
1/2 teaspoon sea salt
1/4 teaspoon black pepper
Dash of cayenne pepper
1/2 teaspoon parsley
1/2 teaspoon basil
1/2 teaspoon oregano
1/2 teaspoon garlic powder
3 pounds (10 slices) thin-sliced chicken breast

Mix the tomatoes, olives, herbs, and spices in a bowl and set aside. Place 5 thin-sliced chicken breasts into an oiled 15 x 10 x 2 Pyrex dish. Add some tomato and olive mixture to each slice. Next, place another 5 thin-sliced chicken breast on top of each of the previously filled breasts. Add the remaining mixture on top of each thin-sliced chicken breast. Place in the oven and low broil for 35 minutes.

Turkey

Preheat oven to 400 degrees F.

Place cut potatoes and place them on the bottom of a large poultry pan with v-shaped rack. Place cut carrots onions on top of the potatoes. Sprinkle with cold pressed olive or sunflower oil, sea salt (small amount), black pepper, and garlic powder.

Place the turkey on the v-shaped rack.

Make a batter of olive or sunflower oil, melted butter (small amount), sea salt (small amount), and black pepper. Inject the batter into the turkey.

Make a "tent" out of aluminum foil and place it loosely over the turkey to keep it moist.

Cook the turkey for 1 hour. Lower the temperature to 350 degrees F.

Insert a cooking thermometer into the breast of the turkey. Cook the turkey until it reaches 165 degrees F. Approximate cooking times:

10 pounds = 3 to 3-1/2 hours
15 pounds = 3-1/2 to 4 hours
20 pounds = 4 to 4-1/2 hours (feeds 10 people)
25 pounds = 4-1/2 to 5 hours
30 pounds = 5 to 5-1/2 hours

Remove the aluminum foil tent 1 hour before the turkey is cooked to brown the skin.

Vegetable Casserole

2 tablespoons cold pressed olive or sunflower oil
2 cloves garlic, chopped
1 onion, chopped (optional)
1 red pepper, chopped
1/2 pound mushrooms, sliced
1 cup lentils, cooked
16 oz. tomatoes, finely chopped
Vegetables, chopped (spinach, bok choy, kale, etc.)
1 teaspoon basil
1/2 teaspoon black pepper
Dash of cayenne pepper
1 teaspoon garlic powder
1 teaspoon oregano
1 teaspoon parsley
1 teaspoon sea salt

    In a 8-quart pot, sauté garlic, peppers, and mushrooms. Add remaining ingredients. Bring to a boil. Cover and simmer for 45 minutes. Serves 6 to 8 people.

Side Dishes

Baked French Fries

Preheat oven 400 degrees F.

4-5 medium sized potatoes, 2 pounds, washed and dried (do not peel).

Okay, they are not fried. But, they taste great and they are healthy too! Wrap the potatoes in wax paper. Cook in a microwave oven for 1.5 minutes on high. Unwrap and insert each potato into the potato slicer creating french fry cuts. Sprinkle rosemary leaves on top. Place the cuts onto a french fry baking sheet (with holes) and bake in a conventional oven for 45 minutes at 400 degrees F or until golden brown or darker if you prefer.

From www.chefscatalog.com

Progressive Deluxe French Fry Cutter, Item # 26027, $34.95

CHEFS Nonstick French Fry Baking Sheet, Item # 29319, $24.95

Broccoli with Tomato Sauce
2 tablespoons cold pressed olive or sunflower oil
2 cloves garlic, chopped
1 onion, chopped (optional)
1 large head of broccoli tips
32 oz. tomato puree
1 teaspoon oregano
1 teaspoon parsley
1/2 teaspoon sea salt
1/8 teaspoon black pepper
1 basil leaf

Sauté garlic in oil. Add garlic and brown. Put all ingredients together in a 6-quart pot. Simmer 30 minutes Serve over rice.

Dahl
1 tablespoon cold pressed olive or sunflower oil
2 cloves garlic, chopped
1/2 cup water or more
1/2 teaspoon black pepper
1/2 teaspoon cardamom
A dash or more of cayenne
1 teaspoon turmeric
1/2 teaspoon coriander
1/2 teaspoon cumin
1/2 teaspoon sea salt
16 oz. lentils

Sauté garlic and oil in a 3-quart pot. Add remaining ingredients. Bring to a boil. Simmer for 30 minutes.

Lentil Salad

Lentils are high in protein and fiber. Fiber will promote bowel movements.

2 cups dry green or brown lentils
4 cups water
1 tablespoon Cold pressed olive or sunflower oil
1/4 teaspoon garlic powder
1/2 teaspoon parsley
1/2 teaspoon basil
1/2 teaspoon oregano
dash of sea salt
dash of black pepper

    Place lentils and water in a 4-quart saucepan. Bring to a boil. Reduce heat, cover, and simmer for 40 minutes or until done. Allow the beans to cool. Then add the remaining ingredients.

Mushrooms in Garlic & Oil

2 tablespoons cold pressed olive or sunflower oil
2 cloves garlic, chopped
1 onion, chopped (optional)
1 pound shitaki or portabello mushrooms, sliced
1 teaspoon parsley
1 teaspoon oregano
1 teaspoon basil
1/2 teaspoon sea salt
1/8 teaspoon black pepper

    Heat oil in a skillet. Add garlic and mushrooms. Sauté until mushrooms and garlic are brown. Add remaining ingredients and sauté another 10 minutes.

Oil and Lemon Dressing

1/4 cup lemon juice (not for migraineur's)
1/2 cup cold pressed olive or sunflower oil
1/2 teaspoon basil
1/2 teaspoon parsley
1 teaspoon oregano
1/2 teaspoon garlic powder
1/8 teaspoon black pepper
1/4 teaspoon sea salt

    Mix all ingredients together in a jar or container. Shake well just before using.

Squash

2 pound butternut squash
2 tablespoons cold pressed olive or sunflower oil
2 cloves of garlic, finely chopped
4 scallions, chopped
1 leek, sliced
1/2 teaspoon sea salt
1/4 teaspoon black pepper
1 pound rice pasta

Peel the butternut squash. Cut the squash into 4 sections length-wise. Remove the seeds. Slice each section into 1/4" slices. Set aside squash. Begin boiling the water for the pasta. At medium heat, add the garlic to a 6-quart pot and sauté until slightly brown. Add the scallions and cook for another minute. Add the leek and cook for another minute. Add the squash and lower heat. Cover and simmer for 20 to 30 minutes or until the squash is tender. Stir occasionally. Serve separately or over pasta or rice.

Steamed Vegetables

6 pieces of broccoli tips
3 slices of cabbage, cut up
2 pieces of kale, cut up
Any additional vegetables you like except potatoes or carrots
1/2 teaspoon basil
1/2 teaspoon parsley
1/2 teaspoon oregano
1/2 teaspoon sea salt
1 tablespoon cold pressed olive or sunflower oil

Place potatoes and cabbage in steamer pot and steam for 15 minutes. Add the rest of the ingredients and steam for an additional 5 minutes. For microwave: cover all vegetables and cook for 10 minutes) Add spices as desired.

Stuffed Artichokes

1 tablespoon cold pressed olive or sunflower oil
2 cloves garlic, finely chopped
6 large-size artichokes
1 teaspoon basil
1 teaspoon parsley
1 teaspoon oregano
1/4 teaspoon sea salt
1/8 teaspoon black pepper

Cut off artichoke stems and trim 1/2 inch from tops of leaves. Separate leaves slightly to allow for stuffing. Sauté garlic and oil until brown. In a large bowl mix together above ingredients. Spoon mixture into the artichokes and place in a steamer pot and steam for 30 minutes at medium heat.

Tossed Salad

Arugula and/or baby spinach
Endive
Radicchio
Garbanzo beans
Oil and lemon dressing

Use quantities of the above appropriate for the number of people being served.

Healthy Gourmet Wheat, Gluten, Dairy, Egg, and Yeast, Free Recipes

Bread and Muffins

Banana Nut Muffins

Preheat oven to 350 degrees F.
2 cups brown rice flour
1 cup tapioca flour
2 tablespoons potato starch flour
2 tablespoons baking powder (non-aluminum)
2 tablespoons fructose or 4 tablespoons sugar
2 teaspoons xantham gum
1/2 teaspoon agar agar
1/2 teaspoon sea salt
4 medium fresh almost green bananas, peeled & mashed
3/4 cup almonds or walnuts, chopped
1-3/4 cups rice or coconut or other milk or water
2 tablespoons cold pressed sunflower oil
1 teaspoon vanilla flavor (non-alcoholic)

    Mix dry ingredients with electric mixer. Slowly add the milk while mixing. Add canola oil and vanilla. Add bananas. Spoon mixture into an oiled muffin pan. Bake at 350 F for 45 minutes or until top is light brown. Remove muffins from the pan and cool on a cake rack. Makes 12 muffins.

Blueberry Muffins

Preheat oven to 350 degrees F.

2 cups brown rice flour

1 cup tapioca flour

2 tablespoons potato starch flour

2 tablespoons baking powder (non-aluminum)

3 tablespoons fructose or 6 tablespoons sugar

2 teaspoons xantham gum

1/2 teaspoon agar agar

1/2 teaspoon sea salt

1-3/4 cups rice or coconut or other milk or water

2 tablespoons cold pressed sunflower oil

1 teaspoon vanilla flavor (non-alcoholic)

1 cup blueberries or other fruit

    Mix dry ingredients with electric mixer. Slowly add the milk while mixing. Add canola oil and vanilla. Add blueberries. Spoon mixture into an oiled muffin pan. Bake at 350 F for 40 minutes or until top is light brown. Remove muffins from the pan and cool on a cake rack. Makes 9 muffins. Add a little water to the unused muffin spaces.

Brown Rice Bread

Preheat oven to 350 degrees F.
2 cups brown rice flour
1 cup tapioca flour
2 tablespoons potato starch flour
2 tablespoons baking powder (non-aluminum)
2 tablespoons fructose or 4 tablespoons sugar
2 teaspoons xantham gum
1 teaspoon agar agar
1/2 teaspoon sea salt
1-1/4 cups rice or coconut or other milk or water
1 tablespoon cold pressed olive or sunflower oil

      Mix dry ingredients with dough hooks. Slowly add the milk while kneading. Add olive or sunflower oil. Dough will be slightly sticky. Press into an oiled loaf pan with a lightly oiled spatula. Bake at 350 F for 60 minutes or until top is medium brown. Remove from the pan and cool on a cake rack. Variations, add 2 teaspoons of Italian seasoning or other seasoning to your taste.

Brown Rice Foccacia Bread

Preheat oven to 400 degrees F.

1 cup brown rice flour

1/2 cup tapioca flour

1 tablespoon potato starch flour

1 tablespoon baking powder (non-aluminum)

1 tablespoon fructose or 2 tablespoons sugar

2 teaspoons xantham gum

1/2 teaspoon agar agar

1/4 teaspoon sea salt

3/4 cup rice or coconut or other milk or water

1/2 tablespoon cold pressed olive or sunflower oil

2 cloves garlic, pressed

    Mix dry ingredients with dough hooks. Slowly add the milk while kneading. Add olive or sunflower oil. Dough will be slightly sticky. Press into an oiled 8-inch baking pan with a lightly oiled spatula. Brush top with olive or sunflower oil. Add garlic, salt, pepper, oregano, fresh basil, thinly sliced tomato. Bake at 400 F. for 25 minutes or until crust is medium brown. Remove from the pan and cool on a cake rack.

Corn Muffins

Preheat oven to 350 degrees F.

2 cups yellow corn meal

1/2 cup brown rice flour

1/2 cup tapioca flour

2 tablespoons potato starch flour

2 tablespoons baking powder (non-aluminum)

3 tablespoons fructose or 6 tablespoons sugar

2 teaspoons xantham gum

1/2 teaspoon agar agar

1/2 teaspoon sea salt

1-3/4 cups rice or coconut or other milk or water

2 tablespoons cold pressed sunflower oil

1 teaspoon vanilla flavor (non-alcoholic)

1 cup corn kernels (optional)

    Mix dry ingredients with electric mixer. Slowly add the milk while mixing. Add canola oil and vanilla. Add optional corn kernels. Spoon mixture into an oiled muffin pan. Bake at 350 F for 40 minutes or until top is light brown. Remove muffins from the pan and cool on a cake rack. Makes 9 muffins. Add a little water to the unused muffin spaces.

Desserts

Almond Cookies and Pancakes

Preheat oven to 350 degrees F.
3 cups or cashew almond flour
1 cup cashew nuts - coarsely chopped
1/2 cup sesame seeds
2 teaspoons baking powder (non-aluminum) (2 tablespoons for pancakes)
2 teaspoons ground cinnamon
1 teaspoon ground nutmeg
1/2 teaspoon sea salt
1/2 cup cold pressed sunflower oil
2 teaspoons xantham gum
1/2 teaspoon agar agar
1/4 cup water (1/2 cup for pancakes)
Organic butter to spread

Mix dry ingredients, then add liquids & mix well. Spoon out onto a lightly oiled cookie sheet with a tablespoon or medium size ice cream scoop. Then, flatten slightly. Bake 30 minutes or until slightly brown. Cool on a wire rack. Makes approximately 26 cookies. Turn the cookie upside down and add butter. 7.6 Carbohydrates per cookie (35 g).

Apple Cashew Dessert

3 medium peeled and sliced apples (390 grams, 50.9 grams carbohydrate)
1-1/4 cups filtered water
1 cup cashew nuts (139 grams, 39.7 grams carbohydrate)
1 cup cashew flour (107 grams, 30.6 grams carbohydrate)
4 tablespoons unsweetened shredded coconut (2.3 grams carbohydrate)
4 fresh organic strawberries, sliced
Cinnamon

     Place all ingredients into a 4-quart saucepan and cook at medium heat for 10 minutes or until the apples are soft. Place the mixture into four 8 oz pyrex cups. Place one sliced strawberry on top of each cup. Sprinkle cinnamon on top of each cup. Refrigerate and serve cold.

     Carbohydrate contents = 130.4 grams divided by 4 = 32.6 grams per serving.

Carrot Cake

Preheat oven to 350 degrees F.

2 cups brown rice flour

1 cup tapioca flour

2 tablespoons potato starch flour

2 teaspoons xantham gum

1 teaspoon agar agar

2 tablespoons baking powder (non-aluminum)

2 teaspoons cinnamon

1 teaspoon salt

1 cup fructose or 2 cups sugar

1/2 cup almonds, chopped

1 cup shredded coconut

2 cups carrots, grated

1 cup cold pressed sunflower oil

1 3/4 cups or more of rice or coconut or other milk

3 teaspoons almond extract

    Combine dry ingredients together. Add liquid ingredients and mix. Add a little water if the mixture is too dry. Put into a 9 x 9 inch oiled pan and bake at 350 F for 45 minutes.

Carob or Chocolate Brownies or Cake

Preheat oven 350 degrees F.
2 cups brown rice flour
1 cup tapioca flour
2 tablespoons potato starch flour
2 tablespoons baking powder (non-aluminum)
2 teaspoons xantham gum
1 teaspoon agar agar
1-1/4 cups carob or chocolate powder (not for migraineur's)
1 cup shredded coconut
1 cup carob or chocolate chips (not for migraineur's)
1/2 teaspoon sea salt
1 cup walnuts or almonds, coarsely, chopped
2 tablespoons cold pressed sunflower oil
1/2 cup fructose or 1 cup sugar
2 teaspoons vanilla flavor (non-alcoholic)
2 cups or more of rice or coconut or other milk or water

Mix dry ingredients. Add liquid ingredients and mix well for a slightly loose mixture. Pour into an oiled 10 x 15 Pyrex baking pan and spread evenly. Bake 40 minutes. Allow to cool completely. Cut into squares and remove from baking dish.

Cashew Cookies and Pancakes

Preheat oven to 350 degrees F.

3 cups cashew flour

1 cup cashew nuts - coarsely chopped

1/2 cup sesame seeds

2 teaspoons baking powder (non-aluminum) (2 tablespoons for pancakes)

2 teaspoons ground cinnamon

1 teaspoon ground nutmeg

1/2 teaspoon sea salt

1/2 cup cold pressed sunflower oil

2 teaspoons xantham gum

1 teaspoon agar agar

1/4 cup water (1/2 cup for pancakes)

Organic butter to spread

     Mix dry ingredients, then add liquids & mix well. Spoon out onto a lightly oiled cookie sheet with a tablespoon or medium size ice cream scoop. Then, flatten slightly. Bake 30 minutes or until slightly brown. Cool on a wire rack. Makes approximately 26 cookies. Turn the cookie upside down and add butter. 8.5 Carbohydrates per cookie (35 g).

Coconut Icing

1/2 cup cold pressed sunflower oil

1/2 cup rice or coconut or other milk

2 tablespoons fructose or 4 tablespoons sugar

1-2 cups shredded coconut (to make thick)

In a blender, mix all ingredients on high for 3 minutes. Apply to the cake with a spatula.

Pie Crust

Preheat oven to 350 degrees F.

1 cup yellow corn meal

1/4 cup brown rice flour

1/4 cup tapioca flour

1 tablespoon potato starch flour

1 teaspoon baking powder (non-aluminum)

2 tablespoons fructose or 4 tablespoons sugar

2 teaspoons xantham gum

1 teaspoon agar agar

1/4 teaspoon sea salt

1/2 cup rice or coconut or other milk or water

3 tablespoons cold pressed sunflower oil

1/2 teaspoon vanilla flavor (non-alcoholic)

Mix dry ingredients with electric mixer. Slowly add milk while mixing. Add canola oil and vanilla. Press into an oiled baking pie plate with a lightly oiled spatula. Add filling and bake at 350 F for 50 minutes or until crust is light brown. Allow to cool completely before serving.

Pie Filling - Apple

2 large apples, peeled and sliced
3/4 cup water
1 teaspoon lemon juice (not for migraineur's)
1 teaspoon cinnamon
1/2 teaspoon nutmeg
2 teaspoons agar agar

    Cover and simmer on low heat for 2 minutes. Add to pie crust.

Pie Filling - Blueberry

16 oz blueberries
3/4 cup water
2 teaspoons agar agar

    Cover and simmer on low heat for 2 minutes. Add to pie crust.

Pumpkin Pudding or Pie Filling

2 cups pumpkin or squash, cooked
1/4 cup fructose
1 teaspoon vanilla flavor (non-alcoholic)
1 teaspoon cinnamon
1/2 teaspoon nutmeg
1/2 teaspoon ground ginger
1/4 teaspoon ground cloves
2 teaspoons agar agar
1 cup rice or coconut or other milk or water

    Simmer ingredients in a 4-quart pot. Stir until mixture is well blended. Pour into pyrex cups, then refrigerate. If used as a pie filling, you do not need to simmer the mixture – add to pie crust.

CPSIA information can be obtained
at www.ICGtesting.com
Printed in the USA
LVHW082140201119
638059LV00018B/1117/P